# The Path To Motherhood

## Birth: Know Your Options

By: Taylor Gilliland

# Disclaimer

**This book is for informational purposes only. Readers are encouraged to confirm the information with other sources. Review this information with your professional health care provider. This book is not intended to replace medical advice offered by physicians.

# Table of Contents:

- - Vacuum
    - C-Section
    - vBac
- What are my options for pain management?
    - Medicated
        - Epidural
            - Standard
            - Walking
        - I.V Medication
        - Nitrous Oxide
    - Natural
        - Water
        - Hypnobirthing
        - Changing position/movement
        - Aromatherapy
        - Massage/pressure
        - Sterile saline injections
        - Birthing ball
        - Hydration
        - Heat Compress
        - Breathing Exercises
- What position can I give birth in?
    - Semi-seated with support
    - Birthing bar
    - Birthing stool

- o Kneeling
  - o Sitting Upright
  - o Side-curled position
- What are the stages of Labor?
  - o 1st Stage
  - o 2nd Stage
  - o 3rd Stage
- Conclusion

*For all moms, everywhere.*

## *Intro:*

———————————

Finding out you're pregnant can fill you with so many emotions: excitement, nervousness, and fear. These are all normal responses. When I was a first-time mom, I too, felt many of those same feelings. I didn't know where to start with getting a provider or what birth would look like for me. I thought I would give birth just like everybody else, and I did. I just went along with whatever my doctor told me to do.

After finding out I was expecting our second baby, I began researching, reading any book or article I could get my hands on. I was determined to be better prepared for the birth of my next child. What I found shocked me. I did not know that I had so many options! I did not have to give birth on my back, numb from the waist down! I had no idea there was more than one way to give birth, more choices for pain management, or that I even had any options at all. I couldn't believe it!

Through my extensive research, I have found that there is no one size fits all, textbook way to give birth. Mothers have options and should be informed so they can make decisions and be prepared. I put this book together to inform mothers who think there is only one way. I hope this book helps you determine the best path for you and your birth.

# Chapter 1

---

## *Where Will I Have My Baby?*

Today in America, most women birth their babies at their local hospital, but it hasn't always been this way. In fact, up until 1940, most births were performed at home. By 1969 less than 1% of births were in an out-of-hospital setting. Hospital births have been the go-to ever since, but that doesn't mean you have to birth your baby in one. There are more places to choose from, although hospitals are a popular choice. When deciding on the setting, take into consideration each one has its own set of pros and cons.

## Hospital Birth

To see if a hospital birth is right for you, schedule a walk through with the one of your choice. They will guide you through the whole labor and delivery ward. The delivery room, the postpartum room, nursery, etc That way you can get a feel of the environment, and so they can answer all your questions and concerns. If you are high risk your doctor, or Midwife may advise you that hospital birth is the best option for you.

<u>*Pros:*</u>

- **Medical Personnel:**
You are surrounded by many medical professionals. If there is an emergency, you are already in the right place to be taken care of. They have the expertise and all the equipment needed to take care of you and your baby if something occurs.

- **Pain Medicine:**
If you do not want to go the natural route and do it without medicine, then a hospital is your best option. They have anesthesiologists' and nurses at the ready to give your pain medicine of choice.

- **Meals:**
I know not everyone loves hospital food, but they do give you three meals a day. This allows you to rest and bond with your baby.

- **Extra Supplies:**
Most hospitals make sure you have everything you need while you are there: Pads, dermasol spray, perineal bottle, formula, nipple cream, diapers, wipes, and bottles. They also send a small package home with you.

- **Nursery:**
I know not all moms want their baby to leave the room, but if you had a difficult birth and need an hour or so of rest, the nursery is there for you to utilize. Use it if you need to.

<u>*Con*:</u>

- **Hard to rest:**
Medical personnel are frequently in and out through all hours of the day and night, the bed is not very comfy, and you are not in the comforts of your own home.

- **Vaccines:**
Whether you decide to vaccinate your child or not, that is up to you, the nurses and doctors will push you to give your child vaccines, plus vitamin K and eye drops. That can be frustrating for parents who do not want to vaccinate when each nurse or doctor that enters the room brings it up repeatedly.
**If you would like to vaccinate your child, then this would be a pro for you. Your nurse can have them ready for you if you wish.

- **Can't go home right away:**
When you deliver at a hospital, the doctor usually wants you and

the baby to stay for at least 1-2 nights. You can not go home until your OBGYN and Pediatrician gives you and baby the all-clear.

- **Not having the freedom to labor and deliver how you would like:** This depends on your doctor and which hospital you use. Some hospitals and doctors will not let you labor or deliver how you would like to. There are more ways to labor and deliver than just laying on your back. Speak to your doctor about this if it is a concern for you. You should be able to freely move about while in labor, unless there is a concern for you or your baby, and push in any position you feel comfortable in.

## Home Birth

Homebirth is perfect for the mom who wants to go all-natural and do it in the comfort of her home. It takes you back in time, to where you can deliver your babies as your great grandmothers and grandmothers did before you. It is quite different than hospital birth. You will be delivering your baby in your home, an environment you are already accustomed to. You will need a Midwife for this. (Please do NOT try and have an unassisted birth! It is dangerous for you and your baby.) You may not qualify for a home birth if you are high risk. Schedule an interview with each midwife you think may be an option to ask them questions to determine which one may be the right fit for you.

<u>Pros:</u>

- **Control:**
  You can control how you labor and deliver your baby. If you want to walk around through contractions, then pop a squat, and push the baby out, you can. It's your choice.

- **Less Hospital Staff:**
  There will only be your midwife
  and maybe 1 assistant with her.
  You won't have to worry about a
  room full of nurses or students
  walking in during your birth.

- **Comfortable:**
  You will be more relaxed because
  you are in the comforts of your
  own home. Also, no hard hospital
  bed.

- **Faster labor:**
  When you are relaxed, and in a
  familiar environment, labor may
  progress faster for you.

- **Home Checks:**
  Your midwife, or her assistant, will
  come to check on you and your
  baby at home for up to 48 hours,
  or more if need be.

<u>*Cons*</u>

- **Not Equipped For Emergencies:**
  If an emergency arises, your midwife may not be equipped to handle it. She will have to call 911 and have you transported to the hospital. This is why high-risk patients are not accepted to do Home Births.

- **No Pain Medication:**
  Most midwives do not offer pain medications. However, in a few states, some midwife practices have started to offer gas and air (laughing gas) as an option for pain.

- **No Nursery:**
  There is no nursery to send your baby to if you need a rest.

- **No prepared meals:**
  Your midwife does not bring you 3 meals a day while you are

recovering like you get when you are in a hospital. You will have to prepare your food yourself unless your partner or a family member does it for you.

## Birthing Center

A birthing center is a more home-esque place to have your baby. It is family-oriented, and they do not use standard interventions. They let your body do what it's designed to do in labor. The Pros and Cons of having your baby at a birthing center are similar to having your baby at home. It could be a good option for those of you stuck between home birth and hospital birth. Call and make an appointment to tour their facility and ask the midwives questions to see if a birthing center is a right fit for you.

<u>*Pros*</u>

- **Comfort:**
Birthing Centers are designed to make you feel comfortable and at home. The rooms are private and lowkey. There is usually no more than two women in labor during the same month, so there is less confusion and more time to make sure your labor and delivery go how you would like it to.

- **Cost:**
The cost of having your baby at a birthing center or home birth is cheaper than a hospital. Prenatal care plus delivery at a birthing center ranges between $2500 to $3000, depending on your state, whereas a hospital could charge you between $8000-$15000.

- **Quick Discharge:**

Birthing Centers usually discharge you somewhere between 6-12 hours after delivery as long as everything went well.

- **Hospital Affiliation:**
  There are two types of birthing centers: free-standing and hospital affiliated. Hospital-affiliated birthing centers are great if you are worried about an emergency arising. They work closely with the hospital and are ready to transfer you quickly to a full team that is waiting for you.

- **Close Proximity to Hospital:**
  Birth Centers are usually located within 10-15 minutes of the closest hospital in case emergencies arise, making it easier to get you to a hospital quickly.

- **Control:**

Just like a home birth, a birthing center gives you the option to labor and deliver how you would like. You have the freedom to go through this beautiful moment in your life, in a manner that is most comfortable for you.

### *Cons:*

- The cons for a birthing center are pretty much the same as having a home birth: **Potentially not equipped for emergencies, no prepared meals, no nursery, and no pain medications.** (besides gas & air, which is offered in some birthing centers)

---

# Chapter 2

# Who WIll Deliver My Baby?

Who will deliver your baby and where you deliver your baby go hand in hand. For example, if you would like to have a home birth, then you would need some form of Midwife. An OBGYN could not be your doctor. This section will teach you a little about each professional who has the knowledge to deliver your baby. 6 different experts have the skills:

## #1) Nurse Practitioner

An OGNP (Obstetric Gynecology Nurse Practitioner) has to receive their Master's in Nursing and pass board exams before they are allowed to begin their career. OGNPs can manage patient visits and ultrasounds but are not allowed to deliver babies unless they continue their education to receive a Certified Nurse Midwife Certification. They must take their CNM Certification test within eight years of graduation to keep from having to complete a midwifery education program. Their CNM certification is valid for three years, and then they can recertify. OGNPs can deliver your baby in any setting; hospital, home, office, etc., but most deliver in a hospital setting. They may not perform a c-section or take on high-risk pregnancies because it is out of their scope of practice.

## #2) OBGYN

An OBGYN (Obstetric Gynecologist) has to obtain a 4-year graduate degree, four years of med school, four years as a resident with a focus in

Obstetrics and Gynecology, and pass the American Board of Obstetrics and Gynecology exam before they begin practicing. They must take a maintenance exam every six years to keep their license. OBGYNs can deliver babies, do surgeries, and treat diseases of the female reproductive organs. They typically deliver babies in a hospital setting but can be on standby at a birthing center should problems arise.

## #3) Maternal-Fetal Medicine Specialist

A MFM (Maternal-Fetal Medicine) is an OBGYN who has completed an additional 2 to 3 years of education and specialized training. They are trained to handle high-risk and non-routine pregnancies. MFMs can not only care for the mother but also, your baby in utero if they need surgeries or support to keep them inside the womb longer. They deliver babies only in a hospital setting.

## #4) Certified Nurse Midwife

A CNM (Certified Nurse Midwife) must obtain a Master's degree in Nursing or higher, graduate from a midwifery education program, have verification from the program director of completion of the education program, and pass the American Midwifery Certification Board Exam (AMCB). They must recertify every five years. CNMs can deliver babies in all settings, but just like Nurse Practitioners, they can not perform C-sections or take on high-risk pregnancies because it is out of their scope of practice.

# #5) Certified Midwife

A CM (Certified Midwife) must obtain a graduate degree from an accredited college or university, complete required health and science classes, and skills training before or within a midwifery program. CM's have to complete the midwifery education program and pass the American Midwifery Certification Board Exam (AMCB). They must recertify every five years. Just as CNMs, CMs can deliver babies in all settings, but they also can not perform C-sections or take on high-risk pregnancies because it is out of their scope of practice.

# #6) Certified Professional Midwife

A CPM (Certified Professional Midwife) is not required to obtain a graduate degree before taking the National

Certification exam. There are no
specified requirements for entry
to the North American Registry of
Midwives (NARM) Portfolio
Evaluation Process (PEP)
apprenticeship. The
apprenticeship must last at least
two years, and they have to assist
with a minimum of 55 births in 3
different categories. CPMs may
obtain a Midwifery Bridge
Certificate to show they meet the
standard minimum education.
They can deliver babies in homes,
birth centers, and offices. CPMs
must recertify every three years.
They can not prescribe medicine,
handle high-risk pregnancies, or
perform c-sections because it is
out of their scope of practice.

---

# Chapter 3

# Do I Need A Birth Partner?

A birth partner is there to support your decisions and coach you through your labor and delivery. It is very helpful to have a birth partner to accompany you during this difficult time. It could be your spouse, a relative, a friend, or a doula.

## _Doula_

A Doula is well trained and has gone through vigorous programs and training to learn how to help and support a mother through pregnancy, labor, delivery, and postpartum. They are a wealth of information and are at your disposal to find out or inform you of all things pregnancy, delivery, postpartum, and baby related. They surpass just being able to help with labor and delivery. Their scope of work is broader.

A Doula can cost you between $250-$1000 depending on your location. It could be more if you require extra services that are not included in their packages. Some Doulas obtain extra certifications so they can further assist you with things you might need, for example: Placenta encapsulation, lactation consulting, prenatal yoga, childbirth education classes, birth photography, etc.

## *Other Non-Professional Partners*

If your spouse, friend, or relative would like to be your birth partner and assist you during labor and delivery, I would recommend they do a little research. There is a wonderful book written by Penny Simkin called, " The Birth Partner: A Complete Guide to Childbirth for Dads, Doulas, and All Other Labor Companions." It is very informative and will have your birth partner educated on what to expect and what you may need from them during that precious time. As long as your birth partner has done research and planned ahead of time to be prepared, then they will do great. If after they have read the recommended book and they feel they are not up to the task, simply ask someone to fill their position, or consider hiring a Doula Service.

# Chapter 4

---

## What Are The Different Types Of Birth?

All babies are not born the same way. Just like every pregnancy is different, so is each birth. Many contrasting outcomes can occur during this time. Some births are planned, some not, and some change in the moment. In this chapter, we will go over the different birthing possibilities.

### <u>Vaginal</u>

Vaginal birth has two options: Natural and Normal.

- In *natural birth,* the mother opts out of all medicated pain options and has no medical intervention, or artificial hormones. The mother has more control over her body and the staff is focused on mom and her wishes and needs.

- A birth is considered a *"normal birth"* if labor starts spontaneously, and the baby is born through the birth canal (vagina).

## Assisted Deliveries

If during a vaginal delivery, the mother is having a hard time birthing the baby, a doctor can use 1 of 2 assisted delivery methods; forceps or a vacuum.

- Forceps: They are two very large, spoon-shaped, metal instruments that are used to cradle the baby's head to help pull and guide the baby out.

- Vacuum: This is not a household vacuum. It is a medical birthing tool that provides suction to the top of the baby's head to help pull and guide the baby out.

These two methods are only used in an emergency if the mother can not get the baby out on her own.


## Water Birth

*Waterbirth* is considered a natural birth. The mother is submerged in a birthing pool filled with warm water, once she reaches about 5cm, for delivery. Her belly should be under the water. A birthing partner can also get into the pool with you for support.

## Induction

When the birth process is started artificially to begin labor and delivery, that is considered induction. It can be used in emergencies or as an elective so you can schedule the child's birth around your schedule. Doctors do not recommend induction for non-medical emergencies, but some doctors do still induce for elective purposes.

There are 2 different types of induction methods:

1.  Medications:
    - Pitocin and Syntocinon: These brand name medications are a form of *oxytocin* the hormone your body naturally creates to stimulate contractions. They are given intravenously.

    - Prostaglandin: These artificial hormones come in the form of capsules, tablets, gels, and suppositories. They are inserted into the vagina to help start labor by softening the cervix and causing uterine contractions.

2. Artificial rupture of membranes:

- Doctors might consider "breaking your water" to speed up labor. They insert a small thin hook inside your cervix to puncture the bag and cause the amniotic fluid to be released. This causes your body to increase the production of prostaglandin, which will speed up your contractions.

## <u>C-Section</u>

A *C-Section ( cesarean)* is used when circumstances will not allow the mother to birth the baby through the vagina. It is a surgical procedure where the baby is born through incisions in the abdomen and uterus. Some women will request to have a non-emergency c-section to have the convenience of a planned birth. This is not recommended because of the potential complications. If you plan on having multiple children, you should know that usually, if you have one c-section, doctors want you to continue to have c-sections for any subsequent pregnancies. With each scheduled c-section you are put more at risk for many complications such as *placenta accreta,* where the placenta abnormally attaches to the muscle of the uterus. It is a very serious complication that can be fatal to the mother. If any way possible, try not to schedule a c-section unless it's needed for your health or an emergency.

## *VBAC*

A VBAC (*vaginal birth after cesarean)* can sometimes be done if your doctor thinks you are a good candidate. If you have one or more of the following risk factors your doctor might not let you try for a VBAC: obesity, pre-eclampsia, older in age, c-section less than 19 months ago, a very large baby, or a previous vertical c-section scar. If you have very little, to no risk factors and have a low horizontal cut, you would be a good candidate. Check with your hospital to see if they are equipped to handle a vbac because not all hospitals are.

*Chapter 5*

---

# *What are my options for pain management?*

Pain management is one of the main topics among mothers. A lot of women think you only have two options: epidural or natural childbirth, that is not true. There are two main categories when researching pain relief options: Medicated and Natural. In this chapter, we will be going through the numerous different methods you can use to get relief during labor and delivery.

## <u>Medicated</u>

- **Epidural:** An epidural is the most popular choice and is used 50% of the time. It is regional anesthesia that blocks feeling from the waist down.

  - **Standard:** A local anesthetic is used to numb the area on your spine then a needle will be inserted between the spine and a catheter put in its place. Medicine will be administered either periodically or continuously. You will not be able to move the lower half of your body at all. You will likely have to receive a catheter for urination so that you can relieve yourself during labor. After the birth of your baby, the epidural catheter will be removed, and feeling should return immediately. However, be very careful walking afterward. You could still have some effects from the epidural for a short time.

- Walking: A walking epidural is very similar to the standard epidural. The only difference is after the catheter is placed between the spine, smaller amounts of medication is administered allowing mom to still move around and not have all feeling taking away. It provides enough pain relief to leave mom comfortable and still able to feel contractions.

- I.V Medication: Only 16% of mothers use i.v meds for pain relief. There are many different pain medications to choose from, but the three most commonly used are stadol, demerol, and nubain. They are administered through an IV port or by intramuscular injection. These medicines may make you feel drowsy so, you can rest. You may not be able to walk around depending on your doctor's recommendations or your hospital's policy.

- **Nitrous Oxide:** Also known as laughing gas, nitrous oxide is an inhaled gas that is slowly making a come back in the U.S. It is estimated that 6% of women in the united states use it during labor and delivery.  It is the same medication used in the dental offices but at a lower strength. Dental offices use the strength of 70/30, where labor and delivery uses a 50/50 blend. It is administered through a hose and face mask. The mom would place the mask over her nose and mouth and breathe during or in between contractions. It does not take the pain away, but it does work in keeping you calm by keeping your panic and anxiety down during labor and delivery. Please check with your hospital to see if they offer this as an option because although it is making a comeback, it still is not available everywhere.

<u>Natural</u>

- Water: Laboring in warm water can help ease the intensity of your contractions, reducing your labor pain or need for pain medication. Floating in between contractions helps you to relax and conserve your energy.

- **Hypnobirthing:** It is a combination of visualization, relaxation, and deep breathing exercises that helps you concentrate on your body and what it needs to do during labor. Hypnobirthing can help you manage stress hormones to help make an easier labor and birth. Stress slows your body's production of oxytocin, and oxytocin is needed to progress labor.

- **Changing Position/Movement:** Changing positions and continuing to move through contractions help reduce the pain of labor. Movement helps move the baby down into the pelvis to get into position.

- **Aromatherapy:** It is the practice of using essential oils from plants to enhance your well being. The oils can be massaged into your skin, added to a warm bath, or diffused into the air. It reduces your stress hormones and in turn, helps you relax and concentrate on labor and delivery.

- **Massage/Pressure:** There are many different methods of applying massage and pressure during labor. Every mother and pregnancy is different, so all methods might not work for everyone. The following are recommended methods of massage and pressure techniques: gentle pressure, kneading, stroking, counter pressure, and reflexology. (the process of massaging and applying pressure to certain parts of the feet to stimulate nerve endings)

- **Sterile Saline Injections:** Saline is injected in small amounts in 4 different locations on your lower back to help reduce back pain during labor. It will not stop the pain from your contractions, but it will help alleviate the pain in your back, which is helpful if you are experiencing back labor. The injections feel similar to a wasp or bee sting, and as the stinging eases, you will begin to feel pain relief in your back.

- **Birthing Ball:** It can ease the discomfort of laboring contractions and put you in comfortable positions to get counter-pressure applied, massages, and help align the spine and pelvis. Here are 4 ball positions you can use with your birthing ball to alleviate the pain of labor: rocking, leaning against the ball, leaning against the ball on all fours, and bouncing. These are just some positions that can help you. Let your body guide you into your most comfortable position.

- **Hydration:** It is very important to stay hydrated during labor. Not being adequately hydrated could result in maternal exhaustion and more likely to need medical intervention. Most hospitals will not allow you to eat or drink during labor but will allow you to suck on ice chips or they can administer i.v. fluids. The uterus functions the best when it is fully hydrated. If it is lacking hydration, it will not work as well as it should, could prolong your labor, or make labor pain worse.

- **Heat Compress:** Using a heat compress can reduce labor pain and also lower your anxiety, helping you to relax. Warm compresses increase the skin temperature arousing the pain receptors in that area relieving pain and making the tissue more flexible. One study shows heat compresses reduce labor pain while also shortening labor time.

- **Breathing Exercises:** Breathing exercises lower your anxiety and panic. They keep you focused on the end goal. Your body will release fewer stress hormones(cortisol) and more pain-relieving hormones(endorphins), helping you stay calm.

---

# Chapter 6

# *What position can I give birth in?*

There are numerous positions that you can use to birth your baby. Here we will talk about 6 of those positions. The best pose to give birth in is the one you are most comfortable in. There is no wrong position as long as you are safe, not in any discomfort(other than labor pains), and not arching your back. The best components of any birthing position is having knees to chest, legs spread, chin tucked down, and hips curled inward to help the baby follow the curves of the pelvis.

Try getting into some of these positions as a practice to see which ones are most helpful for you. Keep in mind, while practicing, you do not want to practice the pushing, but just the

actual position and what does
and does not make you
comfortable.

- **Semi-seated with support:**
  This position is most widely
  used by mothers, especially
  in hospitals. It is not the best
  option, as far as opening
  the pelvis, but it is the most
  used and convenient for
  your doctor. You lie on your
  back with your head and
  shoulders slightly elevated,
  with your legs in stirrups.
  Reach for your legs and pull
  yourself into them, bringing
  your knees closer to your
  chest.

- **Birthing Bar:** A birthing bar
  is an attachment to use on a
  birthing bed that gives
  support in the squatting
  position. It is a great help in
  opening the pelvis and
  using gravity to assist the
  baby down into the birthing

canal. The foot of the bed
drops, allowing you to raise
the head of the bed and use
the bed as a resting chair.
When you feel a contraction
coming, grab the bar and
pull yourself into the
squatting position. After the
contraction is over lean
back onto the head of the
bed to rest.

- **Birthing Stool:** A birthing
  stool is very similar to sitting
  on a toilet, but the front is
  open to catch the baby, and
  it is lower to the ground.
  This position flexes your
  legs and expands the size of
  your pelvis, while gravity
  assists in bringing the baby
  down into the birthing
  canal.

- **Kneeling:** Giving birth on
  your hands and knees is an
  effective position to help
  with back labor pain. You

can do this position on a bed with the head raised or on the floor with pillows for comfort and support, whichever suits you.  While on your hands and knees, lower your butt and flex your hips when you are ready to push. Rest on your forearms with the support of a partner in between contractions to keep your wrists from getting tired.

- **Sitting Upright:** This position is very similar to the birthing stool, where your hips are flexed, and your pelvis is opened while in a sitting position. The bed is set up in the same manner as when birthing with a birthing bar, with the head raised and the foot of the bed dropped down. In this pose sit on the edge of the bed and make sure to tuck your chin and curl forward as you push your baby out. In between contractions, do not forget to lean back and rest either on a partner or the head of the bed.

- **Side-curled position:** This position is best for resting, especially if your labor is unusually long. Lay on whichever side is most comfortable for you and then grab your opposite leg behind the knee and pull it to your chest, opening your pelvis and flexing your hips.

# Chapter 7

---

## What Are The Stages Of Labor?

This is the exciting part! It's almost time for baby's arrival, and you are ready for it to vacate so you can breathe, eat, and not pee every 5.3 seconds! You may be wondering when or what labor will feel like, or what the process is like. Labor and delivery are broken down into 3 stages: Early labor and active labor, delivery of your baby, and delivery of your placenta. I will break down each stage for you so you can get a better understanding of what will happen. Being educated will help you know what to expect.

### _Stage 1:_

Stage one, you will begin to feel regular contractions that will start to open your cervix. It is broken down into 2 separate categories; Early Labor and active labor.

<u>Early Labor:</u>

During early labor, you will start to feel contractions. As your uterus is tightening, you will feel menstrual-like cramps in your abdomen and/or your lower back. You may also notice a light pink bloody discharge from your vagina, indicating that you are starting to lose your mucus plug. Early labor is unpredictable and can last from hours to days. Try to keep your mind busy by doing non-strenuous activities such as walking, meditating, changing positions, or doing laundry. Try to rest as much as possible to get ready for active labor.

<u>Active Labor:</u>

During active labor, your contractions are stronger and last longer. Your cervix is opening between 6 and 10 cm. This stage usually takes hours, but every birth is different. So, it's possible it could last minutes, hours, or days. Try to keep calm and stay positive as best you can. Ask your nurse if you can have intermittent monitoring so that you can move around and try different things to make you comfortable and get through contractions. The last part of this stage is *transition,* this is when your baby moves into the birth canal to get ready to be birthed. This is the most intense part. You will feel a lot of pressure on your lower back and rectum, and your contractions will be longer and more intense than before.

## <u>Stage 2:</u>

Stage two is the birth of your precious bundle of joy. It could take minutes or hours to push your baby into this world. The contractions will be further apart at this stage, giving you time to rest in between pushes. With each push your one step closer to feeling your baby *crown,* It's when the baby's head reaches the perineum causing it to bulge out and making the head visible. You will feel a burning and tingling sensation, some mothers describe it as the ring of fire. As the head emerges out, it will turn to allow the baby's shoulders to rotate to get in position for the final push.  After the baby is pushed out, it will be dried off and placed directly on your chest for skin to skin bonding and to be kept warm.

## Stage 3:

This final stage of labor is the birth of the placenta. It lasts minutes up to an hour. You will be asked for a final push to expel the placenta. It's at this time your doctor will decide to put in any stitches if you happened to tear or needed an episiotomy during birth. There will be a numbing agent before the stitching. This is a walk in the park compared to just having pushed out a baby, don't worry! Your nurses will check on you periodically to make sure you're feeling ok and to push on your abdomen to make sure your cervix is hard.

# *Conclusion*

Women everywhere deserve to know that giving birth does not have to look like what movies depict as the "right way" to bring a baby into the world. You can give birth at home, in the hospital, or at a birthing center; decide to receive pain medication or manage your pain other ways; birth laying on your back or feel free to move about and push in whatever position is most comfortable. Unless medically necessary, whatever you decide, know that there is no wrong answer! Take control of your birth and settle on a plan of action that best suits your wants and needs. When it is all said and done, and you are lying there soaking up your new baby and its new baby smell, bask in the moment. Wear that mom afterglow proudly! Every hard decision you will make to get to that point will be worth it. Labor and delivery

will be over, but your future decisions
and adventures with your little one will
just be beginning.